While every precaution has been taken in the preparation of this book, the publisher assumes no responsibility for errors or omissions, or for damages resulting from the use of the information contained herein.

CONTROL YOUR HEALTH THRU MIND AND BODY

First edition. October 21, 2023.

ISBN: 979-8223681564

Written by Kobus Fourie.

Also by Kobus Fourie

Strange Facts and Wonders
20 Beddie Buy Stories For Kid's
Animals by the Alphabet
Stop That Bad Smoking Habit
Drop Those Extra Pounds
Lyric's For Everyone
Prophecy Revealed
The Intergalactic Quest
My Songs Your Songs
Beyond the Veil
A Life Unveiled: One Man's Journey, Every Person's Story
Savour the Alphabet: 26 Letters, 78 Flavours
The Second Coming Of Jesus
The Timeless Library
Control Your Health Thru Mind and Body

Control Your Health Thru Mind and Body

The mind and body is an intriguing combination and Doctors, Psychiatrists and Specialists have studied it for many years and still they cannot understand it fully.

In this book we will explore this phenomena of Mental Health in the next 4 categories.

- The Mind-Body Connection how to Achieve Emotional Wellness
- Overcoming Anxiety and Strategies for a Calmer Life
- Mindfulness for Everyday Living
- Resilience to Building Mental Strength in a Chaotic World

Kobus Fourie

DEDICATION

Dedicated to all those who strive to nurture their well-being, find strength in resilience, and embark on the journey to a healthier mind and body. May this book inspire and empower you to take control of your health and lead a life of balance and vitality.

CONTENTS

ACKNOWLEDGMENTS

I would like to express my heartfelt gratitude to the following individuals and sources of inspiration who have been instrumental in the creation of this book:

My Family: To my family, who have been my unwavering support system throughout this journey, thank you for your patience, encouragement, and understanding. Your love and belief in me have been my guiding lights.

My Wife: To my beloved wife, who has stood by me with unwavering love and strength, thank you for your constant encouragement and for being my source of inspiration in leading a balanced and healthy life.

My Kids: To my children, for the joy and laughter you bring into my life, and for teaching me the importance of health and well-being through your bright eyes and boundless energy.

Friends: To my friends, old and new, who have shared their stories, experiences, and wisdom. Your camaraderie and support have added depth and richness to the tapestry of this book.

Personal Experiences: To the challenges and triumphs in my own life, you have provided invaluable lessons in resilience and the mind-body connection. Thank you for being my teachers and motivators.

Mentors and Teachers: To those who have shared their expertise and knowledge in the fields of health, well-being, and resilience, your guidance has been invaluable.

Readers and Seekers of Wellness: Lastly, to you, the readers, who have embarked on this journey with me, seeking knowledge and inspiration to enhance your health and well-being. It is my hope that this book will serve as a source of empowerment and guidance on your path to a healthier and more balanced life.

Thank you all for your contributions, support, and presence on this meaningful journey.

The Mind-Body Connection How To Achieve Emotional Wellness

Chapter 1

Understanding the Mind-Body Connection

In the intricate tapestry of human existence, the relationship between our emotional and mental states and our physical health is an integral thread. This profound connection forms the cornerstone of our overall well-being. Welcome to the world of the mind-body connection, a concept that has fascinated thinkers, healers, and scientists throughout history. In this introductory chapter, we will delve into the essence of this connection, exploring how our emotions, thoughts, and physical health are inextricably intertwined.

The Interwoven Fabric of Our Being

Imagine your body as a vast ecosystem, each organ, cell, and molecule working together in perfect harmony. Your emotions and mental state, on the other hand, are the conductors of this symphony, influencing every aspect of your physical being. The mind-body connection is the bridge that links these seemingly distinct domains.

For centuries, medical practitioners and scholars have observed how emotional and mental well-being can either bolster or undermine our physical health. Hippocrates, the father of modern medicine, famously stated, "It is more important to know what sort of person has a disease than to know what sort of disease a person has." In these words, he alluded to the intricate relationship between our emotional state and physical health.

The Science Behind the Mind-Body Connection

Modern science has provided us with a wealth of evidence supporting the existence and significance of the mind-body connection.

CONTROL YOUR HEALTH THRU MIND AND BODY

The field of psychoneuroimmunology, which examines the interaction between our psychological processes, the nervous system, and the immune system, has shed light on how emotions and mental states impact our physical well-being.

The brain, often considered the command centre of our body, plays a pivotal role in this connection. It produces a cascade of chemicals and neurotransmitters in response to our emotional and mental states. For instance, when we experience stress, the brain releases cortisol, commonly known as the stress hormone. Elevated cortisol levels can weaken the immune system, making us more susceptible to illness. Conversely, positive emotions like happiness and love trigger the release of endorphins, which have a multitude of health benefits, from reducing pain to boosting the immune system.

Furthermore, our thoughts and emotions can have a profound impact on our autonomic nervous system. This system governs involuntary bodily functions like heart rate, digestion, and respiratory rate. Through the mind-body connection, we can consciously or unconsciously influence these functions. Deep breathing and relaxation techniques, for instance, can slow the heart rate and promote a state of calm, while anxiety can do the opposite, increasing the heart rate and heightening tension.

The Mind-Body Connection and Health Outcomes

Now, let's consider the real-world implications of the mind-body connection on our health. Numerous studies have shown that individuals with high levels of emotional well-being tend to experience better physical health outcomes. They have stronger immune systems, quicker recovery times from illness, and an increased overall life expectancy. On the flip side, chronic stress, anxiety, and depression can weaken the immune system, exacerbate inflammation, and lead to a range of health issues, including cardiovascular disease and autoimmune disorders.

One of the most compelling aspects of this connection is its ability to influence our ability to heal. The placebo effect, for example, demonstrates the mind's capacity to affect physical healing. When individuals believe they are receiving treatment, even if it's a sugar pill, their bodies can exhibit real improvements. This phenomenon highlights the power of the mind to contribute positively to the healing process.

The Mind-Body Connection in Daily Life

Understanding the mind-body connection empowers us to make informed choices about our emotional and mental well-being, ultimately influencing our physical health. Recognizing the impact of stress, we can proactively engage in stress-reduction techniques such as mindfulness, yoga, or meditation. By fostering emotional intelligence and resilience, we can enhance our ability to cope with life's challenges.

Furthermore, our dietary and exercise choices can be seen through the lens of the mind-body connection. When we nourish our bodies with a balanced diet and engage in regular physical activity, we not only support our physical health but also promote emotional well-being. The release of endorphins during exercise and the nutritional support for brain health through a healthy diet are clear examples of this connection in action.

Chapter 2

The Power of Emotional Intelligence

In the grand tapestry of human experience, emotions are the vibrant threads that weave through every aspect of our lives. They colour our perceptions, shape our interactions, and influence our decisions. But what if we could unravel the intricacies of these emotions, understand them better, and ultimately harness their power for greater emotional wellness? This is where the concept of emotional intelligence (EQ) comes into play, offering us a roadmap to navigate the complex terrain of our feelings and relationships.

Understanding Emotional Intelligence (EQ)

Emotional intelligence, often abbreviated as EQ, is the ability to recognize, understand, manage, and effectively use your emotions as well as the emotions of others. It's a multifaceted skill that encompasses self-awareness, self-regulation, empathy, and social skills. EQ provides us with the tools to navigate the often turbulent waters of our emotional lives with finesse and wisdom.

Self-Awareness: The Foundation of Emotional Intelligence

Self-awareness is the cornerstone of emotional intelligence. It's the ability to recognize and understand your own emotions, including their triggers, intensity, and impact on your thoughts and behaviour. With self-awareness, you become better acquainted with your emotional landscape, allowing you to make conscious choices about how to respond to various situations.

To develop self-awareness, start by simply paying attention to your emotions. Ask yourself how you're feeling in different moments and why. Journaling your emotions can be a valuable practice, enabling you to track patterns and identify what situations or thoughts trigger certain feelings. The goal is not to judge your emotions but to understand them.

Self-Regulation: The Art of Emotional Control

Once you've grasped the landscape of your emotions, the next step is self-regulation. This involves managing your emotions, particularly the more challenging ones, in a way that is healthy and constructive. It's about being able to soothe yourself when upset, control impulsive reactions, and adapt your emotional responses to various situations.

Self-regulation can be practiced through techniques like deep breathing, mindfulness, and meditation. It's also important to identify healthy outlets for your emotions, such as talking to a trusted friend, engaging in creative activities, or engaging in physical exercise. The key is to ensure that you respond to your emotions in a manner that doesn't harm your overall well-being.

Empathy: Understanding the Emotions of Others

Empathy is the ability to recognize and understand the emotions of others. It's a fundamental component of emotional intelligence because it enables us to connect with people on a deeper level. By empathizing with others, we not only enhance our relationships but also broaden our own emotional understanding.

To cultivate empathy, practice active listening. When someone shares their feelings with you, make a conscious effort to understand their perspective, even if it differs from your own. Ask open-ended questions and show genuine interest in their emotional experiences. Empathy is about acknowledging the validity of someone else's emotions, even if they don't align with your own.

Effective Communication: Bridging Emotional Gaps

The final component of emotional intelligence is effective communication. This involves the ability to express your emotions clearly and respectfully while also being receptive to the emotions and perspectives of others. Effective communicators can navigate difficult conversations, resolve conflicts, and build stronger, more harmonious relationships.

To enhance your communication skills, start by being a good listener. Practice active listening by giving your full attention to the speaker, asking clarifying questions, and validating their emotions. When expressing your own feelings, use "I" statements to communicate your emotions without blaming or accusing others. Effective communication is a skill that can be honed through practice and self-reflection.

Emotional Intelligence in Daily Life

The power of emotional intelligence extends far beyond the realm of personal development. It influences our interactions at work, in our families, and in our communities. By honing our EQ, we become more effective leaders, partners, parents, and friends.

In the workplace, leaders with high emotional intelligence can create a more harmonious and productive environment. They understand the needs and concerns of their team members, foster open communication, and resolve conflicts with finesse.

In personal relationships, emotional intelligence enhances our ability to connect on a deep and meaningful level. It allows us to navigate conflicts more effectively, offer support when needed, and strengthen the bonds with our loved ones.

Chapter 3

Stress Management and Resilience

In the complex symphony of our lives, stress is often the discordant note that threatens to overpower the melody of well-being. Stress, in moderation, can be a natural response to life's challenges, motivating us to adapt and grow. However, when it becomes chronic or overwhelming, it can erode our emotional wellness and disrupt the delicate balance of the mind-body connection. In this chapter, we will explore the significance of stress as a factor in this connection, delve into strategies for managing stress, building resilience, and developing effective coping mechanisms.

The Impact of Stress on the Mind-Body Connection

Stress is a fundamental component of the mind-body connection. When we experience stress, whether it's due to work pressures, relationship issues, or external factors, our bodies respond with a "fight or flight" reaction. This response involves the release of stress hormones, such as cortisol and adrenaline, which prepare our bodies for action.

In the short term, this stress response can be helpful. It can increase alertness and focus, helping us address the immediate challenges we face. However, when stress becomes chronic, these constant surges of stress hormones can take a toll on our bodies. Over time, chronic stress can weaken the immune system, elevate blood pressure, and increase the risk of various health conditions, including cardiovascular disease, anxiety, and depression.

Strategies for Managing Stress

The good news is that there are effective strategies for managing stress and mitigating its impact on our emotional and physical well-being. Here are some practical approaches you can incorporate into your daily life:

1. **Mindfulness Meditation:** Mindfulness meditation is a

powerful technique for managing stress. It involves focusing your attention on the present moment, acknowledging your thoughts and feelings without judgment. Regular mindfulness practice can reduce stress, anxiety, and promote emotional well-being.

2. **Physical Activity:** Exercise is a natural stress reliever. It helps to release endorphins, the body's natural mood elevators. Engaging in regular physical activity not only reduces stress but also boosts your overall sense of well-being.

3. **Deep Breathing:** Deep, diaphragmatic breathing can trigger the body's relaxation response. Whenever you're feeling stressed, take a few moments to breathe deeply and slowly. It can calm your nervous system and provide immediate relief.

4. **Progressive Muscle Relaxation:** This technique involves systematically tensing and relaxing different muscle groups in your body. It's a fantastic way to release physical tension that often accompanies stress.

5. **Time Management:** Learning to prioritize tasks and manage your time effectively can reduce the feeling of being overwhelmed. Create a schedule, set realistic goals, and allocate time for self-care.

6. **Positive Lifestyle Choices:** Your diet and sleep patterns play a significant role in stress management. A balanced diet and adequate sleep are essential for emotional and physical well-being. Reducing caffeine and alcohol intake can also help.

Building Resilience

Resilience is the ability to bounce back from adversity, to adapt in the face of challenges, and to develop a greater sense of emotional strength. Resilient individuals are better equipped to cope with stress and maintain their overall well-being. Here are some key factors in building resilience:

1. **Positive Self-Image:** Cultivate a positive self-image by acknowledging your strengths and achievements. This positive self-perception can boost your confidence and resilience.
2. **Social Support:** Build a network of supportive relationships. Friends and family can provide emotional support during stressful times, and sharing your feelings can help alleviate stress.
3. **Problem-Solving Skills:** Enhance your problem-solving skills to tackle life's challenges more effectively. Developing a problem-solving mind set can empower you to take constructive action when facing stressors.
4. **Adaptive Thinking:** Train yourself to view stressful situations with a more positive outlook. Adaptive thinking helps reduce the emotional impact of stress and fosters resilience.

Coping Mechanisms for Resilience

Coping mechanisms are the strategies we use to deal with stress and adversity. They are essential tools for building resilience. Here are some healthy coping mechanisms to consider:

1. **Emotional Expression:** Express your feelings through creative outlets like art, music, or writing. This can be a therapeutic way to process emotions.
2. **Social Connections:** Talk to a trusted friend, family member, or therapist when you're feeling stressed. Sharing your thoughts and emotions can provide comfort and support.
3. **Journaling:** Writing down your thoughts and feelings in a journal can help you gain clarity and perspective on the sources of your stress. It's a valuable tool for self-reflection.
4. **Time Management:** Effective time management can reduce stress by allowing you to prioritize tasks and allocate time for relaxation and self-care.

Chapter 4

Nutrition, Exercise, and Emotional Health

Imagine your body as a finely tuned instrument, and nutrition and exercise as the keys that play a melodious tune. Just as a well-nourished plant thrives and flourishes, your emotional wellness is profoundly influenced by what you consume and how you move. In this chapter, we will explore the essential role of nutrition and physical activity in emotional well-being, highlighting the foods, nutrients, and exercise routines that foster a positive mind-body connection. Additionally, we will provide guidance on how to create a holistic, healthy lifestyle that supports emotional wellness.

The Nutritional Path to Emotional Wellness

Nutrition is the fuel that powers our bodies and minds. It plays a fundamental role in the delicate dance of the mind-body connection. To support your emotional wellness through nutrition, consider these key elements:

1. Balanced Diet: A balanced diet includes a variety of foods from all food groups, providing essential nutrients that support your emotional health. This includes fruits, vegetables, lean proteins, whole grains, and healthy fats. A diverse diet ensures that your body receives the vitamins and minerals it needs to function optimally.

2. Omega-3 Fatty Acids: Omega-3 fatty acids, found in fatty fish like salmon, walnuts, flaxseeds, and chia seeds, are known for their positive impact on emotional well-being. These essential fats help reduce inflammation, promote brain health, and may alleviate symptoms of depression and anxiety.

3. Antioxidant-Rich Foods: Antioxidants, found in foods like berries, dark chocolate, and colourful fruits and vegetables, protect the brain from oxidative stress and inflammation. They are believed to play a role in mood regulation and emotional well-being.

4. Probiotics and Gut Health: Emerging research suggests a strong connection between the gut and emotional health. Fermented foods like yogurt, kefir, and sauerkraut, which contain probiotics, can promote a healthy gut microbiome, potentially influencing mood and stress levels.

5. Hydration: Staying well-hydrated is essential for overall well-being. Even mild dehydration can affect your mood and cognitive function. Drinking enough water throughout the day can help you stay alert and emotionally balanced.

Exercise and Emotional Wellness

Exercise is a powerful tool for enhancing emotional wellness. It doesn't just promote physical health; it also has profound effects on your mood, stress levels, and mental clarity. Here's how exercise can benefit your emotional health:

1. Endorphin Release: Physical activity stimulates the release of endorphins, your body's natural mood boosters. This "feel-good" effect can help reduce symptoms of anxiety and depression and enhance your overall emotional well-being.

2. Stress Reduction: Exercise can act as a stress buster. Engaging in physical activity helps to lower cortisol, the stress hormone, and release tension. Regular exercise can enhance your resilience in dealing with daily stressors.

3. Improved Sleep: Consistent exercise can improve the quality of your sleep, which is vital for emotional wellness. Sleep is the body's natural way of rejuvenating and regulating emotions.

4. Enhanced Cognitive Function: Exercise has been shown to improve cognitive function, memory, and concentration. When your mind is sharp, you are better equipped to manage your emotions and make sound decisions.

5. Social Interaction: Many forms of exercise involve social engagement, whether it's a team sport, group fitness class, or simply walking with a friend. Social interaction is an essential component of emotional wellness, as it provides a sense of connection and support.

CONTROL YOUR HEALTH THRU MIND AND BODY

Creating a Holistic, Healthy Lifestyle

To create a holistic, healthy lifestyle that supports your emotional well-being, it's essential to integrate nutrition and exercise into your daily routine. Here are some practical tips:

1. Meal Planning: Plan your meals with a focus on a balanced diet. Include a variety of colorful fruits and vegetables, lean proteins, whole grains, and healthy fats. Be mindful of portion sizes to maintain a healthy weight.

2. Mindful Eating: Practice mindful eating, which involves savoring your food, eating slowly, and paying attention to hunger and fullness cues. This can help you make better food choices and prevent emotional eating.

3. Regular Exercise: Find a physical activity you enjoy and can maintain regularly. Whether it's walking, swimming, yoga, or dancing, the key is to make exercise a consistent part of your life.

4. Stay Hydrated: Keep a water bottle with you to ensure you drink enough water throughout the day. Dehydration can impact mood and cognitive function.

5. Manage Stress: Use exercise, relaxation techniques, and stress management strategies to address stressors in your life. A balanced diet and regular exercise are also vital components of stress management.

Chapter 5

Mindfulness and Meditation

In the fast-paced and often chaotic world we live in, the art of slowing down and turning our attention inward has become a vital skill for achieving emotional wellness. Enter mindfulness and meditation, two practices that offer a sanctuary of calm amidst the noise of daily life. In this chapter, we will dive into the transformative power of mindfulness and meditation as tools for nurturing emotional well-being. We'll explore how these practices help individuals connect with their emotions, manage stress, and promote mental clarity. Whether you're new to these practices or an experienced meditator, this chapter offers guidance and techniques for all levels.

Understanding Mindfulness and Meditation

Before we delve into the techniques, let's clarify what mindfulness and meditation are:

Mindfulness: Mindfulness is the practice of being fully present in the moment, without judgment. It's about paying attention to your thoughts, emotions, and sensations in a non-reactive way. Mindfulness allows you to observe your inner world as an impartial observer, promoting self-awareness and emotional regulation.

Meditation: Meditation is a technique to achieve a state of deep mental and emotional clarity. It involves focusing your attention on a single point of reference, such as your breath, a mantra, or a visual object. Meditation allows you to enter a state of heightened awareness and inner stillness, promoting relaxation and emotional balance.

The Benefits of Mindfulness and Meditation

Mindfulness and meditation have a host of benefits for emotional wellness:

1. Emotional Awareness: Mindfulness and meditation help you become more attuned to your emotions. By observing your thoughts and feelings, you gain clarity about what's happening within you. This self-awareness is the first step in managing your emotions effectively.

2. Stress Reduction: Mindfulness and meditation are potent stress-reduction tools. They activate the relaxation response in your body, which lowers cortisol levels and helps you deal with stress more gracefully.

3. Emotional Regulation: As you become more aware of your emotions through mindfulness, you can learn to regulate them. Mindfulness enables you to create a gap between stimulus and response, allowing you to choose how you react to emotional triggers.

4. Improved Concentration: Meditation enhances your ability to concentrate and stay focused. This mental clarity can help you manage your emotions and respond to situations with greater equanimity.

5. Enhanced Resilience: Regular mindfulness and meditation practice can boost your emotional resilience. They help you bounce back from adversity more quickly and effectively.

Mindfulness and Meditation for Beginners

For those new to these practices, here are some basic techniques to get you started:

Mindfulness for Beginners:

1. **Mindful Breathing:** Find a quiet place, sit comfortably, and close your eyes. Take a few deep breaths to centre yourself. Pay attention to your breath as it enters and leaves your body. Notice the rise and fall of your chest or the sensation of the breath in your nostrils. If your mind wanders, gently bring your focus back to your breath.

2. **Body Scan:** Lie down or sit comfortably. Start at the top of your head and slowly scan your body, paying attention to any sensations or tension. Breathe into these areas and release tension as you exhale. Move down through your neck, shoulders, and so on, all the way to your toes.

Meditation for Beginners:

1. **Guided Meditation:** Use a guided meditation app or video. Many guided meditations are available for free and provide step-by-step instructions and soothing background music.
2. **Breath Awareness:** Find a quiet place, sit in a comfortable position, and close your eyes. Focus your attention on your breath. Inhale deeply and exhale slowly. If your mind starts to wander, gently bring it back to your breath.

Advanced Techniques:

1. **Loving-Kindness Meditation:** This meditation involves sending well-wishes to yourself and others. It can foster feelings of compassion, empathy, and emotional connection.
2. **Vipassana Meditation:** Vipassana is a traditional Buddhist meditation practice that involves observing the sensations in your body. It can lead to deep insights into the nature of your mind and emotions.

17

Overcoming Anxiety and Strategies for a Calmer Life

Chapter 6

Unraveling the Anxiety Puzzle

Anxiety is an intricate and multi-faceted emotion, one that affects people from all walks of life. It is an emotion experienced by nearly everyone at some point, but when it becomes a constant companion, it can transform into a formidable challenge to emotional well-being. Understanding anxiety's nature and its various forms is the essential first step in overcoming it and crafting a path towards a calmer and more serene life.

The Many Faces of Anxiety

Anxiety is a complex emotional state that manifests in numerous ways. While we often think of anxiety as a feeling of unease or worry, it can present in various forms, including:

1. **Generalized Anxiety Disorder (GAD):** This is characterized by excessive, uncontrollable worry about everyday things. People with GAD often feel anxious without a specific trigger, and their worry can become overwhelming.

2. **Panic Disorder:** Those with panic disorder experience unexpected and intense panic attacks. These attacks can include symptoms such as shortness of breath, heart palpitations, and a sense of impending doom.

3. **Social Anxiety Disorder:** Social anxiety revolves around an intense fear of judgment or scrutiny in social situations. It can be crippling, leading individuals to avoid social interactions.

4. **Specific Phobias:** A specific phobia is an intense and irrational fear of a particular object or situation, such as heights, spiders, or flying.

5. **Post-Traumatic Stress Disorder (PTSD):** PTSD arises after a traumatic event and includes symptoms such as flashbacks, nightmares, and severe anxiety.

6. **Obsessive-Compulsive Disorder (OCD):** OCD involves recurring, distressing thoughts (obsessions) and repetitive behaviours or mental acts (compulsions) aimed at reducing anxiety.

7. **Separation Anxiety Disorder:** This primarily affects children and involves extreme anxiety about separation from loved ones.

The Root Causes of Anxiety

Anxiety is a deeply personal experience, and its root causes can vary widely from person to person. However, several common factors contribute to the development of anxiety disorders:

1. **Genetics:** There is evidence to suggest that genetics can play a role in predisposing individuals to anxiety disorders. If there is a family history of anxiety, an individual may be more susceptible.

2. **Brain Chemistry:** Imbalances in brain chemicals, such as neurotransmitters, can contribute to anxiety. These imbalances affect the brain's ability to regulate mood and emotions.

3. **Life Experiences:** Traumatic events, particularly during childhood, can leave a lasting impact and lead to anxiety. Abuse, neglect, or significant life changes like divorce or loss of a loved one can be triggering events.

4. **Personality:** Certain personality traits, such as perfectionism, a tendency to overthink, or a strong need for control, can make individuals more prone to anxiety.

5. **Medical Conditions:** Some medical conditions and chronic illnesses, as well as the side effects of certain medications, can lead to anxiety symptoms.

6. **Substance Abuse:** Substance abuse, including drugs and alcohol, can exacerbate or lead to anxiety disorders.

Understanding that anxiety can have multiple sources is crucial, as it allows individuals to pinpoint the root causes in their own lives and tailor their approach to managing and eventually overcoming anxiety.

The Journey to a Calmer Life

The road to a calmer and more serene life begins with unraveling the complexity of anxiety. Each person's experience is unique, and there is no one-size-fits-all solution. However, by recognizing the various forms and potential causes of anxiety, individuals can take the crucial first step toward managing and ultimately conquering this challenging emotion.

In the chapters that follow, we'll explore strategies and techniques to address different aspects of anxiety, from managing its symptoms to enhancing emotional resilience. With knowledge and self-awareness, you can begin to chart your path towards a life characterized by inner peace and emotional well-being.

Chapter 7

Taming the Anxious Mind: Practical Techniques

Anxiety often manifests as a torrent of racing thoughts, a mind that refuses to quiet down. But the good news is that there are practical techniques you can employ to regain control and calm your anxious mind. In this chapter, we will explore several proven strategies, including mindfulness, cognitive-behavioral techniques, and relaxation exercises, that can help you rein in your racing thoughts and find serenity in the midst of anxiety.

The Power of Mindfulness

Mindfulness is a potent tool for taming the anxious mind. It involves being fully present in the moment, without judgment, and observing your thoughts and feelings with a sense of detachment. Here's how you can integrate mindfulness into your daily life:

1. **Mindful Breathing:** Find a quiet space, sit or lie down comfortably, and close your eyes. Take a deep breath, focusing on the sensation of the breath entering and leaving your body. When your mind wanders, gently redirect your attention to your breath.

2. **Body Scan:** In a relaxed position, start at your head and move your attention down, scanning your body for tension or discomfort. Breathe into these areas, releasing any tension as you exhale. Continue down through your neck, shoulders, and so on, until you reach your toes.

3. **Mindful Walking:** Take a leisurely walk in a calm environment. Pay attention to each step, the feeling of your feet connecting with the ground, and the sights and sounds around you. If your mind starts to wander, bring your focus back to the experience of walking.

Cognitive-Behavioural Strategies

Cognitive-behavioural techniques are another effective way to manage anxious thoughts. They help you identify and challenge negative thought patterns that contribute to anxiety. Here's how to get started:

1. **Identify Negative Thoughts:** Pay attention to your thoughts when you're feeling anxious. What are the recurring, distressing thoughts that race through your mind? Write them down.

2. **Challenge Negative Thoughts:** Analyse these thoughts. Are they based on evidence? Are they overly negative or unrealistic? Challenge them with more balanced, rational perspectives. Ask yourself if there is another, more realistic way to look at the situation.

3. **Replace Negative Thoughts:** Once you've challenged your negative thoughts, replace them with more constructive and positive ones. For instance, replace "I can't handle this" with "I can take it one step at a time."

Relaxation Exercises

Relaxation exercises can help soothe the anxious mind and reduce physical tension. Try incorporating the following techniques into your routine:

1. **Deep Breathing:** Inhale deeply through your nose for a count of four, hold for four counts, and then exhale through your mouth for four counts. This simple exercise can trigger the body's relaxation response.

2. **Progressive Muscle Relaxation:** Tense and release different muscle groups, starting with your toes and working your way up to your head. This exercise helps alleviate physical tension.

3. **Visualization:** Close your eyes and imagine a peaceful, calming place. It could be a beach, a forest, or anywhere that makes you feel serene. Picture yourself there and immerse yourself in the details.

Creating a Calming Routine

To fully embrace these practical techniques, consider creating a calming routine. Set aside time each day for mindfulness, cognitive-behavioural exercises, or relaxation techniques. Consistency is key to reining in racing thoughts and calming the anxious mind.

By incorporating these strategies into your daily life, you can begin to regain control over your anxious thoughts and find moments of serenity, even in the midst of anxiety. In the chapters ahead, we'll delve deeper into additional techniques and strategies to enhance your emotional well-being and create a life marked by calm and resilience.

Chapter 8

Navigating Stress and Coping with Triggers

Stress and anxiety often go hand in hand. Stress can be the fuel that ignites anxiety and makes it burn brighter. Understanding stress, its sources, and how to manage it is a critical step in the journey towards overcoming anxiety. In this chapter, we will dissect the various sources of stress and provide strategies to manage and reduce it. Additionally, we'll delve into identifying personal triggers and developing effective coping mechanisms to navigate the turbulent waters of anxiety and stress.

Sources of Stress

Stress can originate from various facets of our lives, and it's essential to recognize where it may be coming from. Common sources of stress include:

1. **Work:** Job-related stress can be triggered by high demands, long hours, conflicts with colleagues, or job insecurity.
2. **Personal Relationships:** Relationship difficulties, whether with a partner, family member, or friend, can be significant stressors.
3. **Financial Concerns:** Money worries, such as debt or financial instability, can lead to chronic stress.
4. **Health Issues:** Managing health problems, whether acute or chronic, can be a source of ongoing stress.
5. **Major Life Changes:** Events like divorce, relocation, or the loss of a loved one can bring significant stress.
6. **Daily Hassles:** Everyday annoyances, like traffic or a malfunctioning appliance, can add to daily stress.

Strategies to Manage and Reduce Stress

Understanding the sources of stress is only the beginning. To manage and reduce stress effectively, consider these strategies:

CONTROL YOUR HEALTH THRU MIND AND BODY

1. **Time Management:** Organize your day, set priorities, and allocate time for tasks and relaxation. Effective time management can reduce feelings of being overwhelmed.
2. **Healthy Lifestyle:** A balanced diet, regular exercise, and adequate sleep are crucial for stress management. A healthy body is better equipped to cope with stress.
3. **Relaxation Techniques:** Practice relaxation exercises, such as deep breathing, meditation, or progressive muscle relaxation, to soothe your nervous system.
4. **Mindfulness:** Incorporate mindfulness techniques into your routine. By staying present in the moment, you can reduce the impact of stressful thoughts and scenarios.
5. **Social Support:** Lean on your support network. Sharing your worries and concerns with friends or family can alleviate stress.
6. **Limit Exposure to Stressors:** When possible, minimize your exposure to sources of stress. For instance, if a particular news source or social media platform consistently raises your stress levels, consider limiting your engagement.

Identifying Triggers and Coping Mechanisms

In addition to managing overall stress, it's essential to pinpoint personal triggers that exacerbate anxiety. Identifying these triggers can help you develop tailored coping mechanisms. Here's how to get started:

1. **Keep a Journal:** Maintain a journal of stressful situations and your emotional responses. This can help you identify patterns and specific triggers.
2. **Self-Reflection:** Engage in self-reflection to uncover your individual triggers. Are there particular situations, people, or thoughts that consistently heighten your anxiety?
3. **Seek Professional Help:** If identifying triggers feels challenging, consider consulting a mental health professional. They can offer insights and guidance.

Once you've identified triggers, work on developing coping mechanisms:

1. **Cognitive Restructuring:** Use cognitive-behavioral techniques to reframe your thinking when faced with triggers. Challenge negative thought patterns and replace them with more positive and rational ones.
2. **Mindfulness and Relaxation:** Practice mindfulness and relaxation techniques when triggers arise. By staying present and calm, you can reduce the emotional impact.
3. **Healthy Distractions:** Engage in hobbies or activities that provide a healthy distraction when faced with triggers.
4. **Social Support:** Reach out to friends or family for emotional support and guidance in dealing with triggers.

By navigating stress and identifying triggers, you can develop a toolbox of coping mechanisms that enable you to manage anxiety effectively. In the upcoming chapters, we'll continue to explore strategies to enhance emotional well-being and create a calmer, more serene life.

Chapter 9

The Power of Self-Care: Emotional and Physical Wellness

Self-care is more than just a buzzword; it's the cornerstone of managing anxiety and nurturing emotional and physical well-being. In this chapter, we'll explore the profound significance of self-care in promoting balance and resilience in your life. From nutrition and exercise to relaxation and nurturing hobbies, you'll discover how to cultivate a lifestyle that not only manages anxiety but also fosters emotional and physical wellness.

The Significance of Self-Care

Self-care encompasses the deliberate actions you take to nurture your physical, mental, and emotional health. It's about recognizing that your well-being is a top priority and taking steps to ensure it remains in balance. The significance of self-care in managing anxiety cannot be overstated. Here's why it's essential:

1. **Stress Reduction:** Self-care activities help you manage and reduce stress, which is often a significant contributor to anxiety. By engaging in relaxation techniques and nurturing practices, you can soothe your nervous system.

2. **Emotional Resilience:** Self-care equips you with the emotional strength to navigate challenging situations and cope with anxiety more effectively.

3. **Physical Health:** Taking care of your physical health through self-care activities, such as regular exercise and a balanced diet, ensures that your body is better prepared to handle the physical effects of anxiety.

4. **Self-Compassion:** Self-care fosters self-compassion, which is crucial for managing anxiety. It encourages you to treat yourself with kindness and understanding, rather than self-criticism.

Nurturing Emotional Wellness

Emotional well-being is at the core of self-care. Here are some strategies to nurture it:

1. **Mindfulness and Relaxation:** Incorporate mindfulness and relaxation practices into your routine to reduce stress and enhance emotional balance.
2. **Emotional Expression:** Express your emotions through creative outlets like art, writing, or music. It's a healthy way to process and release pent-up emotions.
3. **Social Connection:** Cultivate and maintain meaningful relationships. Social support is a vital aspect of emotional well-being.

Prioritizing Physical Health

Physical well-being is intimately connected to emotional health. Here's how to take care of your body:

1. **Nutrition:** Consume a balanced diet rich in fruits, vegetables, lean proteins, whole grains, and healthy fats. Proper nutrition is vital for managing anxiety.
2. **Exercise:** Engage in regular physical activity. Exercise not only promotes physical health but also releases endorphins, which improve mood and reduce anxiety.
3. **Sleep:** Ensure you get enough quality sleep. Sleep is when the body and mind rejuvenate, making it crucial for emotional well-being.

Balancing Work and Life

Finding a balance between work and personal life is an essential component of self-care. Here's how to achieve it:

1. **Set Boundaries:** Establish clear boundaries between work and personal time. Avoid overextending yourself with work commitments.

2. **Take Breaks:** Incorporate short breaks throughout the day to recharge and reduce stress.
3. **Hobbies and Interests:** Nurture hobbies and interests that bring you joy and relaxation. These activities provide an essential escape from the pressures of daily life.

Creating a Self-Care Plan

To make self-care a consistent part of your life, consider creating a self-care plan. This plan outlines self-care activities you can incorporate daily, weekly, or monthly. It might include:

- A daily practice of mindfulness or meditation.
- Weekly exercise sessions.
- Monthly self-care rituals, such as a spa day or a nature hike.

Having a self-care plan provides structure and ensures that you prioritize your well-being regularly.

Chapter 10

Building Resilience and a Calmer Tomorrow

The journey towards overcoming anxiety and achieving a calmer life is a path of growth and self-discovery. In this final chapter, we'll provide you with a roadmap to build resilience, enhance emotional wellness, and ensure a calmer future. You'll learn how to bounce back from anxious episodes, set meaningful goals, and create a life that's filled with serenity and emotional strength.

The Power of Resilience

Resilience is the ability to withstand adversity and bounce back from life's challenges. It's a quality that can be developed and nurtured, and it's crucial for managing anxiety effectively. Here's how to build resilience:

1. **Mindset Shift:** Begin by shifting your mindset. View challenges as opportunities for growth and learning rather than insurmountable obstacles.
2. **Self-Compassion:** Treat yourself with kindness and self-compassion. Understand that setbacks and moments of anxiety are a part of the human experience.
3. **Learn from Adversity:** Reflect on your experiences with anxiety. What have you learned about yourself and your triggers? Use this knowledge to prepare for future challenges.

Setting Meaningful Goals

Goals give you direction and purpose. By setting goals, you create a roadmap for the future and a reason to strive for emotional well-being. Here's how to set meaningful goals:

1. **Identify Values:** Consider what matters most to you in life. Your values are a compass that can guide your goals.
2. **Set SMART Goals:** SMART goals are Specific, Measurable, Achievable, Relevant, and Time-bound. This framework

ensures that your goals are clear and attainable.

3. **Break It Down:** Divide larger goals into smaller, manageable steps. This makes it easier to track your progress and celebrate achievements along the way.

Creating a Calmer Future

To ensure a calmer future, it's crucial to integrate all that you've learned into your daily life. Here are some strategies to help you achieve a serene and emotionally strong future:

1. **Consistency:** Consistency is key. Continue your self-care practices and strategies, even when you start to feel better. Regular self-care can prevent anxiety from resurfacing.
2. **Flexibility:** Life is full of surprises and challenges. Be flexible in your approach to anxiety management. Adapt your strategies as needed.
3. **Embrace Change:** Embrace change as a natural part of life. Change can be an opportunity for growth and adaptation.
4. **Seek Support:** Don't hesitate to seek support from friends, family, or mental health professionals when needed. Building resilience doesn't mean you have to face challenges alone.
5. **Celebrate Progress:** Celebrate your achievements, no matter how small. Recognize and acknowledge your progress in managing anxiety and fostering emotional wellness.

A Calmer Tomorrow

Your journey towards a calmer tomorrow is a testament to your strength and determination. By building resilience and setting meaningful goals, you're actively shaping the future you desire. A calmer life is within your reach, and you have the tools and knowledge to maintain it.

As you move forward, remember that you have the power to overcome anxiety, navigate life's challenges, and cultivate emotional strength. The journey doesn't end here; it's an ongoing process of self-discovery and personal growth. With the insights and strategies provided in this book, you can embrace a future that's marked by serenity, emotional wellness, and resilience.

32

Mindfulness for Everyday Living

Chapter 11

The Essence of Mindfulness

In the hustle and bustle of our modern lives, we often find ourselves lost in the whirlwind of thoughts and distractions. We're consumed by the past, worried about the future, and rarely fully present in the here and now. This is where mindfulness comes into play. In this opening chapter, we embark on a journey to explore the essence of mindfulness, its origins, and the profound benefits it offers for enhancing our everyday existence.

What is Mindfulness?

At its core, mindfulness is the practice of being fully present in the moment, with an open and non-judgmental awareness of our thoughts, emotions, and sensations. It's about cultivating a state of active, focused attention, free from the clutter of the past or the worries of the future. Mindfulness invites us to experience life as it unfolds, savouring each moment with a sense of curiosity and acceptance.

The Origins of Mindfulness

While mindfulness has gained popularity in the West in recent years, it has ancient roots in Eastern philosophies and contemplative traditions. One of the most well-known origins of mindfulness is found in Buddhism, where it's an integral part of the path to enlightenment. Mindfulness meditation, often referred to as Vipassana, has been practiced for thousands of years as a way to gain insight into the nature of reality and the self.

In the modern context, the practice of mindfulness has been secularized and adapted to suit a variety of lifestyles and belief systems. Jon Kabat-Zinn, a pioneer in the field, developed the Mindfulness-Based Stress Reduction (MBSR) program in the late 1970s, which brought mindfulness into the realm of medicine and psychology. This marked a significant turning point in the integration of mindfulness into Western culture.

The Power of Mindfulness

Mindfulness offers a range of benefits that make it a valuable practice for enhancing everyday life. Here are a few of the key advantages:

1. **Stress Reduction:** Mindfulness has been proven to reduce stress by promoting relaxation and improving the body's response to stressors. It helps individuals better cope with the challenges of everyday life.

2. **Emotional Regulation:** Through mindfulness, individuals can develop greater emotional intelligence, becoming more aware of their emotions and learning how to respond to them effectively.

3. **Enhanced Concentration:** Regular mindfulness practice sharpens focus and concentration, which can lead to increased productivity and improved decision-making.

4. **Better Relationships:** Mindfulness promotes empathetic listening, effective communication, and an open-hearted approach to relationships, thereby strengthening connections with others.

5. **Physical Health:** Research has shown that mindfulness can have a positive impact on physical health by reducing symptoms of chronic illnesses, lowering blood pressure, and improving sleep.

Setting the Stage for Your Mindfulness Journey

Your journey into mindfulness begins with a simple yet profound shift in awareness. By recognizing the power of being fully present in the moment and embracing mindfulness, you lay the foundation for a more fulfilling and enriching life. Throughout this book, we'll explore the practical aspects of integrating mindfulness into your daily routine, and you'll learn how to bring mindfulness into various aspects of your life. With each step, you'll move closer to reaping the benefits of this ancient practice in our fast-paced, modern world.

As we continue, we'll delve into practical mindfulness exercises, techniques, and strategies that you can easily incorporate into your daily life. By the end of this journey, you'll have the tools and insights to lead a more mindful, purposeful, and enriching everyday existence. The power to enhance your life through mindfulness lies within your grasp, and it starts with a simple commitment to being present and open to the moment.

Chapter 12

The Practice of Daily Mindfulness

In Chapter 1, we uncovered the essence of mindfulness and its profound potential to enhance our everyday existence. Now, in Chapter 2, we embark on the practical journey of integrating mindfulness into our daily lives. This chapter is your guide to the nuts and bolts of mindfulness, where you'll learn about mindfulness exercises, techniques, and how to cultivate a state of mindfulness in everyday activities. By the end of this chapter, you'll be equipped with step-by-step guidance on how to bring mindfulness to your daily routine.

The Mindfulness Toolbox

To practice mindfulness effectively, it's essential to have a toolbox of techniques and exercises at your disposal. This toolbox allows you to tailor your mindfulness practice to your needs and preferences. Here are some key components:

1. Mindful Breathing:

Mindful breathing is one of the simplest yet most powerful mindfulness exercises. It involves paying full attention to your breath, focusing on the sensation of each inhalation and exhalation. This exercise can be practiced anywhere, at any time, making it an excellent choice for weaving mindfulness into your daily routine.

2. Body Scan:

A body scan involves systematically directing your attention to different parts of your body, from your toes to the top of your head. This exercise helps you become more attuned to physical sensations and can be a great way to relax and release tension.

3. Mindful Eating:

Mindful eating invites you to savour your food fully. It encourages you to eat slowly, paying attention to the taste, texture, and smell of each bite. This exercise not only enhances your connection to food but also helps prevent overeating.

4. Daily Activities:

Everyday activities offer numerous opportunities for practicing mindfulness. Whether it's brushing your teeth, taking a shower, or doing the dishes, you can bring mindfulness into these routine actions. Focus your attention on the sensations and movements involved in these activities.

Cultivating Mindfulness Throughout the Day

Mindfulness is not restricted to formal meditation sessions; it can be cultivated throughout the day. Here's how to integrate mindfulness into your daily activities:

1. Morning Routine:

Start your day mindfully. As you wake up, take a few moments to focus on your breath and set an intention for the day. As you go through your morning routine, such as brushing your teeth or taking a shower, bring your full attention to the sensations and actions.

2. Mindful Commuting:

Whether you drive, bike, or take public transport to work, your commute can be an opportunity for mindfulness. Pay attention to the sights, sounds, and sensations around you. It's a chance to start the day with a sense of presence.

3. Mindful Work:

Integrate mindfulness into your workday by taking short breaks for mindful breathing or mini-meditation sessions. These moments of mindfulness can enhance your focus and reduce stress.

4. Mindful Eating:

Lunchtime is an ideal time for mindful eating. Instead of rushing through your meal, savor each bite, and appreciate the flavors and textures of your food.

5. Evening Wind Down:

As the day comes to a close, create a ritual for winding down mindfully. This could involve a relaxation exercise or mindful breathing to help you transition into a peaceful evening.

Chapter 13

Mindfulness for Stress Reduction

Stress has become an inevitable part of modern life, often affecting our physical and mental well-being. Fortunately, mindfulness offers a powerful antidote to the relentless demands and pressures that surround us. In this chapter, we delve into the transformative role of mindfulness as a tool for managing stress. We'll explore various mindfulness strategies designed to reduce stress, including mindful breathing, meditation, and techniques for staying present amidst life's challenges. By the end of this chapter, you'll have a comprehensive understanding of how mindfulness can be harnessed to navigate the tumultuous waters of stress more effectively.

Understanding Stress

Before we explore how mindfulness can alleviate stress, it's crucial to understand what stress is and how it affects us. Stress is a physiological response to challenging situations, whether they're physical, emotional, or psychological. While a certain amount of stress can be motivating and adaptive, chronic stress can have detrimental effects on our health and well-being. Common stressors include work-related pressures, relationship conflicts, financial concerns, and health issues.

The Mind-Body Connection

The mind-body connection is a crucial aspect of understanding stress and how mindfulness can alleviate it. Stress triggers a physiological response known as the "fight-or-flight" response. When this response is activated, our bodies release stress hormones like cortisol and adrenaline, which prepare us to face a perceived threat. Over time, chronic stress can lead to an array of physical and mental health issues, including anxiety, depression, and heart disease.

Mindfulness for Stress Reduction

Mindfulness offers a pathway to combat the detrimental effects of stress by allowing us to respond to life's challenges with greater resilience and poise. Here are several mindfulness strategies for stress reduction:

1. Mindful Breathing:

Mindful breathing is a foundational mindfulness practice that can be used as a quick stress reduction technique. When you're feeling stressed, take a moment to focus on your breath. Inhale deeply through your nose and exhale slowly through your mouth. This simple exercise can help reduce the body's stress response.

2. Meditation:

Meditation is a more in-depth mindfulness practice that involves sustained, focused attention. Through meditation, you can cultivate a heightened awareness of your thoughts and emotions, making it easier to manage stressors. There are various forms of meditation, such as loving-kindness meditation, body scan meditation, and mindfulness of breath meditation, each with its unique benefits for stress reduction.

3. Staying Present Amidst Challenges:

Mindfulness teaches us to remain present in the face of life's challenges rather than succumbing to the automatic reactions of stress. By observing your thoughts and emotions with non-judgmental awareness, you can choose to respond to stressors with calm and clarity.

4. Mindfulness-Based Stress Reduction (MBSR):

Mindfulness-Based Stress Reduction (MBSR) is a structured program developed by Jon Kabat-Zinn. It integrates mindfulness meditation and mindfulness practices into a comprehensive approach for managing stress, anxiety, and pain. MBSR programs are widely available and can be a valuable resource for those seeking stress reduction through mindfulness.

The Power of Mindfulness

Mindfulness is a transformative practice that can rewire the brain's responses to stress over time. By cultivating mindfulness, you develop emotional intelligence, self-awareness, and the ability to respond to stressors with resilience and composure. Mindfulness enables you to break free from the cycle of stress, allowing you to navigate life's challenges with greater ease.

Incorporating Mindfulness into Your Daily Life

Throughout this chapter, we'll delve deeper into each of these mindfulness strategies and offer practical guidance on incorporating them into your daily life. By the end of this chapter, you'll have the tools to respond to stress with mindfulness and embark on a journey towards greater well-being and emotional resilience. As we progress, you'll find that mindfulness is not just a practice; it's a way of life that empowers you to conquer stress and lead a more balanced and fulfilling existence.

Chapter 14

Mindful Relationships and Communication

In our daily lives, few things have as much impact as the quality of our relationships. Whether it's with our partners, family members, friends, or colleagues, these connections shape our emotional well-being. Mindfulness has a profound role to play in fostering healthier relationships by enhancing our communication, empathy, and the depth of our connections. In this chapter, we'll explore how to integrate mindfulness into your interactions with others, with a focus on fostering better communication, deeper empathy, and stronger relationships. By the end of this chapter, you'll have the tools to listen mindfully, resolve conflicts peacefully, and enrich your relationships.

The Role of Mindfulness in Relationships

Mindfulness provides a powerful framework for understanding and improving relationships. It enables you to be fully present with others, to listen with an open heart, and to respond with compassion and empathy. Here are several key ways in which mindfulness benefits relationships:

1. Better Communication:

Mindfulness helps you become a more attentive and active listener. By staying present in the moment and fully engaging with what others are saying, you can avoid misunderstandings and enhance the quality of your communication.

2. Empathy and Compassion:

Mindfulness fosters a deeper sense of empathy and compassion. When you approach others with an open and non-judgmental attitude, you're better equipped to understand their perspective and respond with kindness.

3. Conflict Resolution:

Mindfulness teaches you to stay calm and composed, even in the face of conflicts. This can be invaluable in resolving disputes peacefully and with respect for one another's feelings and needs.

Applying Mindfulness in Relationships

Here are some practical ways to apply mindfulness in your relationships:

1. Mindful Listening:

Listening mindfully involves giving your full attention to the speaker. Put away distractions, maintain eye contact, and focus on what the other person is saying. Avoid formulating your response while they're speaking, and instead, truly absorb their words.

2. Non-reactive Responses:

When you respond to others, especially in the midst of disagreements or conflicts, do so mindfully. Instead of reacting impulsively, take a moment to breathe and consider your response. Mindful responses are typically more thoughtful and less emotionally charged.

3. Mindful Empathy:

Empathy is about truly understanding and sharing the feelings of others. Practice putting yourself in their shoes and acknowledging their emotions with an open heart. This can be especially helpful in times of distress or when offering support to a loved one.

4. Conflict Resolution:

When conflicts arise, bring mindfulness into the equation. Rather than escalating the situation, create space for open dialogue. Mindful conflict resolution involves listening, acknowledging feelings, and working together to find a solution that respects the needs of all parties involved.

The Power of Mindful Relationships

Mindfulness has the power to transform your relationships by infusing them with deeper connection, empathy, and open communication. When you approach your interactions with mindfulness, you create an environment that fosters understanding, trust, and emotional safety.

Cultivating Mindful Relationships

Throughout this chapter, we'll explore practical exercises and strategies for cultivating mindful relationships. You'll learn how to harness the power of mindfulness to enrich your connections with others and create a more harmonious and empathetic social environment. By the end of this chapter, you'll have the tools to listen mindfully, resolve conflicts peacefully, and strengthen your relationships, all while infusing them with the grace and wisdom of mindfulness. As we move forward, you'll discover that mindfulness is not just a personal practice; it's a cornerstone of harmonious and fulfilling relationships.

Chapter 15

Mindfulness and Everyday Well-being

As we reach the culmination of our journey into mindfulness, it's time to bridge the gap between the practice of mindfulness and its profound impact on your everyday well-being. In this final chapter, we'll connect the dots between mindfulness and various aspects of your life, including mental clarity, emotional balance, and physical health. You'll discover how mindfulness can serve as a guiding light on your path to a fulfilling, balanced, and well-rounded everyday existence.

The Holistic Benefits of Mindfulness

The practice of mindfulness transcends a mere exercise in stress reduction or self-improvement. It's a holistic approach to life that embraces the mind, body, and spirit. Here are some of the holistic benefits of mindfulness:

1. Mental Clarity:

Mindfulness sharpens your mental focus and clarity. By practicing mindfulness, you can enhance your cognitive abilities, including memory and problem-solving. This mental clarity translates into more productive and effective daily activities.

2. Emotional Balance:

Mindfulness equips you with the tools to manage your emotions more effectively. You become better at recognizing and processing your feelings, allowing you to respond with a sense of balance and composure, even in emotionally charged situations.

3. Physical Health:

Mindfulness has been linked to a host of physical health benefits. Regular practice can lead to lower blood pressure, improved sleep, and better immune system function. Additionally, mindfulness can help with chronic pain management and the prevention of stress-related diseases.

4. Increased Resilience:

Mindfulness cultivates resilience, enabling you to bounce back from life's challenges with greater strength. It helps you view difficulties as opportunities for growth and learning, rather than insurmountable obstacles.

Mindful Eating for Better Nutrition

One of the areas where mindfulness profoundly affects everyday well-being is nutrition. Mindful eating is an approach that encourages a conscious awareness of the foods you consume and how they affect your body. By paying full attention to the process of eating, you can make more informed food choices, avoid overeating, and foster a healthier relationship with food.

Enhancing Physical Health through Mindful Movement

Mindful movement practices, such as yoga and tai chi, are another way in which mindfulness enhances physical well-being. These practices involve the integration of breath, movement, and focused attention, promoting flexibility, strength, and balance. They also serve as excellent tools for stress reduction and relaxation.

Mindfulness for Better Sleep

Quality sleep is a cornerstone of well-being. Mindfulness practices can help you improve the quality of your sleep by calming the mind, reducing stress, and promoting relaxation. Techniques such as mindfulness meditation before bedtime can contribute to a restful night's sleep.

The Journey Towards Everyday Well-being

As we conclude this journey into mindfulness, it's important to recognize that mindfulness is not a destination; it's a lifelong journey. You have the tools and insights to integrate mindfulness into your daily life, and by doing so, you can significantly enhance your well-being. Mindfulness allows you to experience each moment more fully, leading to greater joy, fulfillment, and peace in your everyday existence.

The Power of Mindfulness for Everyday Well-being

Incorporating mindfulness into your daily life means living with intention and presence. You'll find that everyday tasks become opportunities for mindfulness, and as you continue to practice, you'll experience the profound transformation of your well-being. By weaving mindfulness into the fabric of your life, you can achieve greater mental clarity, emotional balance, and physical health. With each mindful moment, you'll enhance the quality of your life and set yourself on a path to a more fulfilling, balanced, and well-rounded existence.

Resilience to Building Mental Strength in a Chaotic World

Chapter 16

Understanding Resilience

In the face of life's uncertainties, adversities, and the chaotic nature of the world we inhabit, resilience stands as a powerful shield and a guiding light. It is a quality that enables individuals not just to endure but to thrive in the midst of challenges. In this opening chapter, we'll embark on a journey to explore the essence of resilience, understanding its significance and the role it plays in building mental strength.

What Is Resilience?

At its core, resilience is the capacity to adapt, bounce back, and even flourish in the face of adversity. It is the ability to withstand stress, setbacks, and overwhelming circumstances, emerging from these experiences stronger, wiser, and more capable. Resilience isn't an innate trait that only a fortunate few possess. It's a skill that can be developed and nurtured, making it accessible to everyone.

Why Resilience Matters in a Chaotic World

In a world characterized by constant change, uncertainty, and unforeseen challenges, resilience takes on profound importance. Here's why resilience matters in navigating a chaotic world:

1. **Coping with Uncertainty:** Chaos often brings uncertainty and unpredictability. Resilience equips you to handle ambiguity and make effective decisions, even in the absence of clear answers.

2. **Bouncing Back from Setbacks:** Chaotic environments are breeding grounds for setbacks and disappointments. Resilience

enables you to recover from these setbacks, learn from them, and maintain your forward momentum.

3. **Adapting to Change:** Resilience is the foundation of adaptability. In a chaotic world, the ability to adapt to shifting circumstances and environments is invaluable.

4. **Mental Strength:** Resilience contributes significantly to mental strength. It helps you manage stress, stay composed in the face of adversity, and preserve your emotional well-being.

The Components of Resilience

Resilience is not a single, monolithic trait but a combination of several components. Understanding these components is the first step in building mental strength. Here are some key elements of resilience:

1. **Emotional Regulation:** Resilient individuals are adept at managing their emotions. They can acknowledge their feelings without being overwhelmed by them.

2. **Optimism:** A positive outlook on life and a belief in the ability to overcome challenges are essential components of resilience.

3. **Problem-Solving Skills:** Resilient individuals are resourceful problem-solvers. They approach obstacles with a mind-set focused on finding solutions.

4. **Social Support:** Strong social connections provide an essential foundation for resilience. A support system of friends and family can be a crucial resource during challenging times.

5. **Adaptability:** The ability to adapt to changing circumstances is a hallmark of resilience. Resilient individuals are flexible and open to new approaches.

Nurturing Resilience

While resilience is partly influenced by genetics and early life experiences, it can be developed and strengthened over time. The journey to resilience is marked by self-awareness, personal growth, and a commitment to building mental strength. Throughout this book, we'll explore practical exercises, strategies, and real-life examples that will help you nurture your resilience.

Chapter 17

The Science of Stress and Coping

Stress is an inherent part of the human experience, and in a chaotic world, its prevalence and impact are profound. In this chapter, we will embark on a journey into the science of stress, understanding its implications for mental health, and the strategies individuals employ to cope with it. By delving into the physical and psychological effects of stress, we'll discover the pivotal role of resilience in managing and even thriving in the face of chaos.

The Nature of Stress

Stress is a physiological and psychological response to demanding situations. When faced with challenges, the body activates its stress response system, releasing hormones like cortisol and adrenaline. This "fight-or-flight" response prepares us to confront or escape perceived threats. While this response is crucial for survival, prolonged or chronic stress can be detrimental to mental and physical health.

Physical Effects of Stress

The physical effects of stress are extensive and can have a significant impact on overall well-being. They include:

1. **Elevated Heart Rate:** Stress can increase heart rate and blood pressure, potentially leading to heart problems over time.
2. **Weakened Immune System:** Chronic stress can weaken the immune system, making individuals more susceptible to illness.
3. **Digestive Issues:** Stress can lead to digestive problems like indigestion, irritable bowel syndrome, and ulcers.
4. **Muscle Tension:** Stress can cause muscle tension and pain, particularly in the neck, shoulders, and back.
5. **Sleep Disturbances:** Stress often leads to sleep difficulties, which can exacerbate mental health issues.

Psychological Effects of Stress

Stress doesn't only affect the body; it also has significant psychological effects. These include:

1. **Anxiety and Worry:** Stress can lead to heightened anxiety, constant worry, and rumination.
2. **Depression:** Chronic stress is a known risk factor for depression, contributing to the development and exacerbation of depressive disorders.
3. **Cognitive Impairment:** Stress can impair cognitive function, affecting memory, decision-making, and problem-solving.
4. **Emotional Dysregulation:** Stress can make individuals more emotionally reactive and less able to manage their emotions effectively.

The Role of Resilience

Resilience acts as a buffer against the adverse effects of stress. Resilient individuals have a greater ability to cope with stress and recover from its impact. They approach challenges with a more positive outlook, seek solutions, and maintain their emotional well-being during difficult times. The key elements of resilience, such as emotional regulation, optimism, and problem-solving skills, all contribute to effective stress coping.

Thriving in the Face of Chaos

The chaos of the modern world is often accompanied by an increase in stressors, from work pressures to personal challenges. However, understanding the science of stress and how to cope effectively is a powerful step toward thriving in this chaotic environment. Resilience is not about eliminating stress, but about developing the capacity to adapt and grow stronger in the face of adversity.

Chapter 18

Developing Resilience Skills

Resilience is not an innate trait; it's a skill that can be developed and nurtured. In a chaotic world, building mental strength and resilience is crucial to not just surviving but thriving. In this chapter, we'll explore practical strategies and exercises designed to enhance your resilience. You'll acquire a toolkit to bolster your mental strength, navigate challenges, and emerge from adversity even stronger.

Cognitive Reframing

One of the most powerful resilience skills is cognitive reframing. It involves changing the way you perceive and interpret challenging situations. Here's how it works:

1. **Identify Negative Thoughts:** When confronted with adversity, identify negative thoughts and beliefs that arise. For example, if you fail at a task, you might think, "I'm a failure."

2. **Challenge and Reframe:** Challenge these negative thoughts by asking yourself if they're truly accurate. In the case of failure, you can reframe it as a learning opportunity: "I can learn from this experience and do better next time."

3. **Cultivate Positive Self-Talk:** Replace negative self-talk with positive and constructive messages. For example, "I can handle this challenge" or "I am resilient."

Stress Management Techniques

Stress management is an essential aspect of resilience. The ability to manage stress effectively is the cornerstone of mental strength. Here are some stress management techniques to consider:

1. **Mindfulness and Meditation:** Mindfulness practices can help you stay present, reduce stress, and enhance resilience. Meditation is an excellent tool for calming the mind and

building emotional regulation.

2. **Breathing Exercises:** Deep breathing exercises can instantly reduce stress. When you feel overwhelmed, take a moment to practice deep, diaphragmatic breathing to calm your nervous system.

3. **Physical Activity:** Regular exercise releases endorphins, which are natural stress relievers. Engaging in physical activity helps manage stress and promotes mental well-being.

4. **Journaling:** Keeping a journal can be a powerful way to process and manage stress. Writing down your thoughts and emotions allows you to gain insight and perspective on challenging situations.

Problem-Solving Skills

Resilient individuals are adept problem-solvers. They approach challenges with a solution-focused mindset. Here's how to enhance your problem-solving skills:

1. **Identify the Problem:** Clearly define the problem or challenge you're facing. Sometimes, identifying the problem itself can be half the solution.

2. **Brainstorm Solutions:** Generate a list of potential solutions or approaches to the problem. Don't censor your ideas; simply let them flow.

3. **Evaluate and Choose:** Evaluate the pros and cons of each solution. Choose the one that appears to be the most effective and feasible.

4. **Take Action:** Once you've chosen a solution, take action promptly. Implementation is a crucial step in effective problem-solving.

Building Social Support

Strong social connections are a cornerstone of resilience. Building and maintaining a support system is vital. Here's how to do it:

1. **Nurture Relationships:** Invest time and effort in your relationships. Maintain connections with friends and family who provide emotional support.
2. **Seek Help:** Don't hesitate to reach out for help when needed. Asking for support is a sign of strength, not weakness.
3. **Offer Support:** Be willing to support others in their times of need. Building a reciprocal support system strengthens bonds and enhances resilience.

Chapter 19

Navigating Uncertainty and Adversity

In a world marked by chaos and rapid change, uncertainty and adversity are ever-present companions on life's journey. This chapter centers on the pivotal role of resilience in helping individuals navigate these challenges. You'll learn how to adapt to change, bounce back from setbacks, and recognize opportunities for growth amidst chaos.

Adapting to Change

Adaptability is a core facet of resilience. It is the capacity to respond effectively to changing circumstances, embrace new realities, and adjust one's approach as needed. Here's how resilience empowers individuals to adapt to change:

1. **Flexible Mindset:** Resilient individuals maintain a flexible mindset. They understand that change is a natural part of life and accept it without resistance.
2. **Positive Attitude:** Resilience fosters a positive attitude toward change. Instead of viewing change as a threat, resilient individuals often perceive it as an opportunity for growth and learning.
3. **Problem-Solving Skills:** Resilience is closely tied to effective problem-solving. When confronted with change, resilient individuals approach it as a problem to be solved, seeking innovative solutions and strategies.

Bouncing Back from Setbacks

Setbacks are an inescapable aspect of life. Resilience equips individuals to bounce back from these setbacks, learn from them, and continue to progress. Here's how resilience helps in this regard:

1. **Embracing Failure as Learning:** Resilient individuals view failure as a valuable learning experience. Instead of dwelling on

the disappointment, they focus on the lessons and insights it provides.

2. **Maintaining Emotional Regulation:** Resilience helps individuals maintain emotional stability even in the face of setbacks. This emotional regulation enables them to approach challenges with composure and determination.

3. **Seeking Support:** Resilient individuals are not afraid to seek support when faced with setbacks. They recognize that reaching out to friends, family, or professionals is a crucial part of bouncing back.

Finding Opportunities for Growth

Resilience enables individuals to perceive opportunities for growth even in the most challenging circumstances. It allows them to extract meaning and wisdom from adversity. Here's how:

1. **Personal Growth:** Resilient individuals often experience personal growth as a result of adversity. They become wiser, more empathetic, and better equipped to face future challenges.

2. **Enhanced Problem-Solving Skills:** Adversity can be a catalyst for improving problem-solving skills. Resilient individuals become more adept at identifying solutions and adapting to change.

3. **Increased Self-Awareness:** Confronting adversity often leads to increased self-awareness. Resilient individuals gain a deeper understanding of their strengths, weaknesses, and values.

Chapter 20

Cultivating Mental Strength for the Long Haul

In the final chapter of our journey on resilience, we'll explore how to sustain and continually strengthen your mental resilience in a world that is ever-changing and often chaotic. The ability to maintain mental strength for the long term is essential for not only surviving but thriving in the face of life's uncertainties. In this chapter, you'll discover strategies for self-care, ongoing learning, and the importance of nurturing your mental strength for sustained well-being.

The Importance of Long-Term Mental Strength

Building mental resilience is not a one-time endeavor but a lifelong journey. Life's challenges don't stop once you've developed resilience; they continue to test and shape your mental strength. Here's why maintaining mental strength for the long haul is crucial:

1. **Adapting to a Changing World:** The world is in a constant state of flux. The ability to adapt and remain mentally strong is vital for navigating ongoing changes.

2. **Coping with Multiple Stressors:** You'll encounter various stressors throughout your life, from work-related challenges to personal setbacks. Maintaining mental strength equips you to cope effectively with these stressors.

3. **Promoting Long-Term Well-being:** Mental strength contributes to long-term well-being. It helps you preserve your emotional health, make positive life choices, and live a fulfilling and meaningful life.

Strategies for Cultivating Long-Term Mental Strength

Here are strategies and practices for nurturing your mental strength for the long haul:

1. Self-Care

Self-care is not a luxury; it's a necessity for maintaining mental strength. Regular self-care practices promote emotional and physical well-being. Consider these self-care strategies:

- **Daily Stress Reduction:** Incorporate daily stress reduction techniques into your routine, such as meditation, deep breathing, or mindful moments.
- **Physical Health:** Prioritize your physical health through regular exercise, a balanced diet, and adequate sleep.
- **Hobbies and Interests:** Engage in hobbies and interests that bring you joy and relaxation.
- **Boundaries:** Set healthy boundaries to protect your time and emotional energy.
- **Rest and Relaxation:** Schedule regular periods of rest and relaxation to recharge.

2. Ongoing Learning

Life is a continuous learning journey, and ongoing learning is crucial for maintaining mental strength. Here's how to embrace lifelong learning:

- **Adaptability:** Develop a growth mindset that embraces challenges and sees them as opportunities for learning and growth.
- **Education:** Pursue ongoing education, whether formal or informal, to expand your knowledge and skills.
- **Resilience Practice:** Continue to practice resilience-building techniques regularly to reinforce your mental strength.

3. Support Systems

Maintaining mental strength often requires the support of others. Cultivate and nurture your support systems:

- **Social Connections:** Stay connected with friends and family members who provide emotional support.
- **Professional Help:** Don't hesitate to seek professional help when needed. Therapists and counselors can offer guidance during challenging times.
- **Peer Groups:** Consider joining support groups or communities that focus on resilience and well-being. Sharing experiences and insights with others can be empowering.

4. Mindfulness and Reflection

Regular mindfulness and self-reflection practices can help you stay attuned to your mental well-being. They allow you to monitor your emotional state, identify areas for growth, and develop a deeper understanding of yourself.

5. Setting and Pursuing Goals

Setting and pursuing meaningful goals can provide a sense of purpose and direction. Goals give you a reason to remain mentally strong and continue to strive for personal and professional growth.

ABOUT THE AUTHOR

Kobus Fourie resides in a tranquil rural town nestled within the picturesque landscape of the Free State, South Africa. His life is enriched by the love of his wonderful wife, his cherished children, and the delightful company of their beloved dogs.

Kobus has always had a passion for writing, and his journey as an author is a testament to this deep-seated love for words. His writing is profoundly rooted in personal experiences, reflecting the genuine authenticity of his life and the insights it has bestowed upon him.

In his small town, amidst the serene countryside, Kobus found inspiration in the everyday moments that often go unnoticed. These ordinary but meaningful experiences have shaped his perspective on health, well-being, and the intricate connection between mind and body.

Kobus's writing is a reflection of his desire to share the wisdom he has gained from his own life's journey. It is an endeavour to inspire and guide others in their pursuit of a more balanced, healthier, and mindful existence. His commitment to storytelling and his unwavering dedication to his craft shine through in the pages of this book.

Kobus Fourie's journey as an author is an embodiment of his personal philosophy — that life's most profound lessons are often hidden in the beauty of the everyday, and that by sharing these experiences, we can all find a path to better health and well-being. This book is a testament to his love of writing and his desire to make a positive impact on the lives of those who read his words.

Don't miss out!

Visit the website below and you can sign up to receive emails whenever Kobus Fourie publishes a new book. There's no charge and no obligation.

https://books2read.com/r/B-A-KVXX-LORPC

BOOKS2READ

Connecting independent readers to independent writers.

Did you love *Control Your Health Thru Mind and Body*? Then you should read *A Life Unveiled: One Man's Journey, Every Person's Story*[1] by Kobus Fourie!

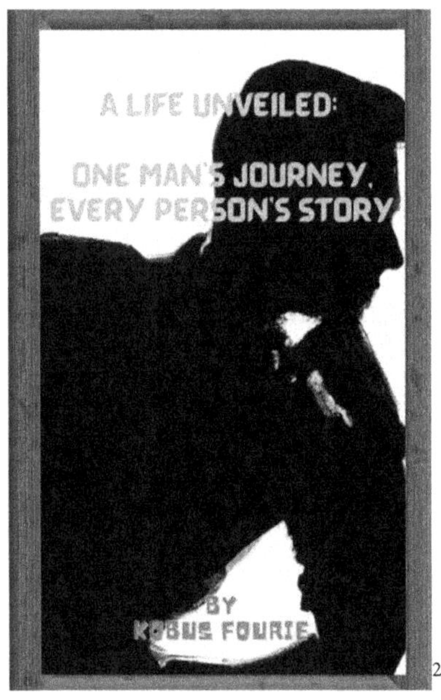

[2]

Explore the remarkable journey of one man through life's twists and turns, a story that mirrors the struggles and triumphs we all encounter. From personal losses and professional challenges to resilience and redemption, this memoir uncovers the shared human experiences that connect us all. Delve into the depths of personal growth, faith, and love as you embark on a transformative odyssey. 'A Life Unveiled' offers a poignant reflection on the beauty and strength found in the midst of adversity, inspiring readers to find hope, courage, and meaning in their own lives.

---

1. https://books2read.com/u/4EpYPe

2. https://books2read.com/u/4EpYPe

Also by Kobus Fourie

Strange Facts and Wonders
20 Beddie Buy Stories For Kid's
Animals by the Alphabet
Stop That Bad Smoking Habit
Drop Those Extra Pounds
Lyric's For Everyone
Prophecy Revealed
The Intergalactic Quest
My Songs Your Songs
Beyond the Veil
A Life Unveiled: One Man's Journey, Every Person's Story
Savour the Alphabet: 26 Letters, 78 Flavours
The Second Coming Of Jesus
The Timeless Library
Control Your Health Thru Mind and Body